A BEGINNERS GUIDE TO ESSENTIAL OILS

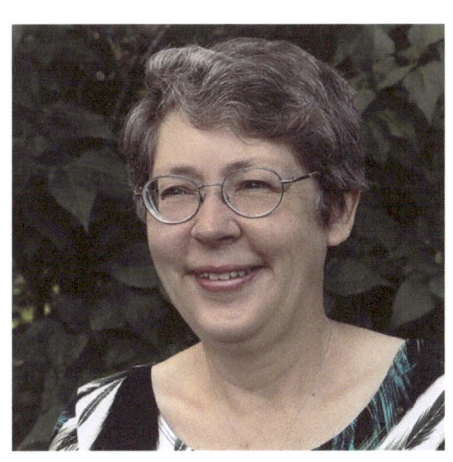

BY: CYNTHIA K. FORCK

CONTENTS

INTRODUCTION

Hello and welcome to my Beginners Guide on Essential Oils. My name is Cynthia and I live in a rural area in Central Missouri. I am a single person who is retired from working for the state for over 30 yrs.

Now I am living my passion of helping people like You learn about organic living and the use of Essential Oils. I put this guide together to help you with the use of Essential Oils.

I have long been a proponent of homeopathic medicine and non-traditional healing as opposed to prescription drugs. Over the years I have discovered a wealth of information about essential oils and their use. In the pages that follow, I intend to pass that knowledge to you

Now law requires me to advise you that I am not a doctor and I cannot diagnose or treat any disease. Before embarking on your journey of self-healing and homeopathy, you should consult your own physician

In the twelve chapters that follow, you will find a plethora of information to guide you in your discovery of the benefits and uses of essential oils.

Peace to You,   *Cynthia*

CHAPTER ONE

THE BEGINNING OF ESSENTIAL OILS

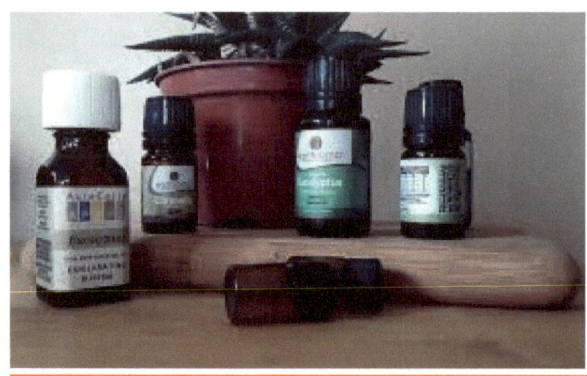

Essential Oils are the oldest form of medicine known to man. God created the seeds, plants and trees before he even created man.

 It is only recently that chemical substances have been used by men. These chemicals are lacking in purity, adding harmful compounds with adverse side effects.

Since ancient times, and as near as we can tell, from the beginning of recorded history the plant kingdom has provided rare and powerful extracts and essences that have long been prized for their beauty enhancing, medicinal, spiritual, aromatic and therapeutic value.

Aromatic plants, essences and oils have been used for ages in ceremony, religious observances, beauty care, food preparation and preservation, as incense, and for perfumes.

Aromatic plants have also been the basis for herbal and botanical medicines and remedies for thousands of years. In fact, they're the root of today's pharmaceuticals.

The earliest essential oils usage evidence occurs in the period of 3000-2500 B.C.

It's common for Egyptians to be given credit as the first culture to use aromatic extracts for beauty care, culinary uses, spiritual and physical wellbeing. But it is believed that essential oil-like extracts were also being used in China and India at nearly the same time. Depending on who is citing historical evidence, you can also find references to Ayurvedic uses of essential oils in India much earlier.

Whichever way we look at it, history of many cultures has enriched and enhanced valuable aspects of the essential oils and aromatherapy world.

CHAPTER TWO

HISTORY OF ESSENTIAL OILS

All throughout history Essential Oils have been used to treat many types of ailments. Ancient Egyptian hieroglyphic and Chinese manuscripts reference the use of Essential Oils to heal the sick. Essential Oils were considered very valuable to many ancient cultures.

During the Dark Ages in Europe many people died from the plague. These fatal epidemics were very contagious, and no one wanted to remove the dead bodies for fear of contacting the illness. However, there were some thieves who would rub a blend of clove, lemon, eucalyptus, cinnamon and rosemary on their bodies and put on masks for breathing. This way they were able to go into the homes of the dead and rob them of their possessions without getting the disease. This combination has a 96% kill rate against bacteria in the air. It has been tested alongside E. Coli and Staph infections and has been just as effective as antibiotics.   This combination can be applied to the soles of the feet without diluting during the cold and flu season. Diffusing in the home is another way to use the combination.

Some ask how could Jesus afford the costly oils? Well, His ministry was underwritten financially by His women followers who He had helped when they were sick. He also had many wealthy friends and followers. Not to mention several of these disciples were affluent. The Holy Land itself was a major producer of essential oils from its own native vegetation. It was a major crossroads of the oil trade of the world. Liquid spices were available and diluted with olive oil. The disciples stretched the oils as for as they could to help more people when anointing the sick. The anointing oils with prayers were very powerful.

One of the oils what was plentiful during that time was cedarwood. The cedar trees were magnificent attaining awesome height and diameters. Some lived to a great old age of 2,000 years. Some of the seedlings in Christ's day may still be alive today. It is thought that inhaling cedarwood enhances the ability to think clearly and can be used for more effective prayer and meditation. It has a high concentration of sesquiterperpenes (98%) and has the ability to pass through the blood brain barrier and help the brain directly upon inhalation by way of the nasal passages and the olfactory nerves. It has been thought that cedarwood oil might prevent senility and Alzheimer's disease.

As early as 2000 BC, the ancient Egyptians were using essential oils for medicinal benefits, beauty care, spiritual enhancement, and in literally all aspects of their daily life.

The Egyptians were passionate about beauty; they took beauty care very seriously and were considered highly accomplished in specialized beauty care treatments. In fact, Cleopatra's legendary beauty is attributed to her extensive use of the customary Egyptian essential oils, fatty oils, clays and salts from the spa on the edge of the Dead Sea – gifted her by Marc Antony, and other naturally occurring treatments.

The Egyptians were the first civilization to distill cedarwood oil. They used it for many things such as emotional clearing, embalming, increasing mental clarity and as an insect repellant. The kings of the time used cedarwood for their homes and temples.

CHAPTER THREE

ESSENTIAL OILS FOUND IN THE BIBLE

Oils were essential to daily living back in Biblical times. In fact the word "oil" appears in the King James Version of the Bible 191 times – more than the words believe, grace and joy!

This doesn't take into account the times generic references like odors, sweet savors, perfumes, balms and ointments were used. It also doesn't include incense burners or even spices, which could include some fragrant herbs. Now, of course, not all of these oil mentions in the Bible were essential oils. The cruder olive oils were used for lighting of their lamps. The first press olive oil was used for cooking and flavoring of foods.

There are some mixed opinions on whether fragranced oils (early versions of essential oils) were truly essential oils or olive oil that was heavily infused with different herbs and plants. Distillation pots have been found as early as 3500 B.C., so it would be possible but no one knows for sure.

Some of these fragranced oils were to make incense. I don't know about you but I used to love incense but most are used with cheap and toxic fragrance chemicals. In fact, some people are concerned that today's incense should never be used in the presence of young children due to its danger!

Ancient incense was very important and sacred and used in many occasions and ceremonies

As stated above, Essential Oils were referred to 191 times in the bible. To "anoint" meant "to smear with oil", to make a person sacred and dedicate them to serve a higher spiritual purpose.

Additionally, a plague was referred to in the bible that was stopped by preparing a sacred temple with aromatic oils. The baby Jesus received Gold, Frankincense, and Myrrh from the 3 Wise men at His birth. Some historians think that the "Gold" referred to a valuable "liquid gold" called Balsam Oil.

The origin of anointing was from the shepherds of the day. Lice and other insects would often get into the wool of sheep, and when they got near the sheep's head, they could burrow into the sheep's ears and kill the sheep. So, ancient shepherds poured oil on the sheep's head. This made the wool slippery, making it impossible for insects to get near the sheep's ears because the insects would slide off. From this, anointing became symbolic of blessing, protection, and empowerment.

The New Testament Greek words for "anoint" are chrio (cree-O) which means "to smear or rub with oil" and, by implication, "to consecrate for office or religious service"; and aleipho (E-life-o), which means "to anoint." In Bible times, people were anointed with oil to signify God's blessing or call on that person's life. A person was anointed for a special purpose—to be a king, to be a prophet, to be a builder, etc.

It is clear that a true Biblical anointing was not a small dot of veggie oil applied somewhere but a true anointing was usually more than that. It was usually a considerable amount of oil.

CHAPTER FOUR

ESSENTIAL OILS AS POWERFUL HEALERS

When you inhale or topically apply a pure essential oil you are inhaling and receiving the essence of the healing plant.

The energy inside the plant combines with the intelligence inside each of us to allow healing to occur.

Essential oils that are produced at a low-quality level or artificially altered have their precious potency forever changed.

Find a company that never alters the essence of the plant.

CHAPTER FIVE

USDA CERTIFICATION

Users of essential oils should be aware that the oil should be USDA Certified Organic. Oils going through the USDA Certification are certified at the point of origin (at the farm) and then again at the distribution level in USA. They are:

- Wild crafted and grown in the wild

- Not produced with commercial farming

- Select farmed -farming that produces therapeutic oils

- Do not have any herbicides or pesticides used on them

CHAPTER SIX

STRICT SOURCING REQUIRED

1. No child labor
2. Must not damage the earth or surrounding community
3. No testing on animals
4. Oils must be USDA certified Organic, wild crafted and free of chemicals
5. Farm and distiller must have through knowledge on the correct time to harvest oils and distill for excellent therapeutic effect. Some oils must be picked only in the morning and then distilled that same morning.
6. No genetically modified organism
7. No artificial colors or scents of any kind
8. Oils must not be mixed with chemical compounds
9. Oils must be teste with GCMS, Gas Chromatography Mass Spectrometry units. This insures that all compounds are present at the correct standard required for a true therapeutic effect
10. Oils either or rejected or approved. This insures proven results to you and every customer.

CHAPTER SEVEN

SAFE GUARDS FOR THE USE OF ESSENTIAL OILS

Essential oils should be used with caution. You can use either vegetable oil or massage oil as a carrier. Mix your carrier oil with your pure essential oil and apply a small amount to your wrist to test for any possible sensitivity or allergy. . If it heats up or turns red, discontinue use of the oil and consult a knowledgeable professional

Everybody's body and emotional makeup are different. If you have allergies or a medical condition, consult a health care professional as well as a knowledgeable essential oils expert.

If the Essential Oils accidentally get in your eyes, you should use liquid vegetable oil. Rub the oil around your eye. Do not use water as that will exaggerate the pain. So the bottom line is: do not use water.

I personally would recommend that you not store the oils near your eye drops so as not to mistake the two when using them.

When any of the citrus oils are used such as Lemon Essential Oil, wait 12 hours before going into the sun. The oil can cause sun burns.

Always, if on medication, check with your physician before the use of Essential Oils because some can interact with medicine.

Are Essential Oils Safe to Use Around My Pets?

Essential Oils that are NOT SAFE for dogs:

• Clove. • Garlic. • Juniper. • Rosemary. • Tea tree. • Thyme. • Wintergreen. ...

Essential Oils that are NOT SAFE for cats: • Cassia. • Cinnamon. • Lemon. • Citrus. • Clove. • Eucalyptus. ...

CHAPTER EIGHT

ANTIOBITICS VS. ESSENTIAL OILS

In the last hundred years, drugs like antibiotics have been produced to treat infections. When an antibiotic is used. billions of bacteria are killed yet one or two survive. These can multiply until there are billions of them that are not affected by the antibiotics.

Drug companies must continually develop new and more powerful antibiotics that can kill the resistant strains. But until a new antibiotic is developed the resistant bacteria can make us sick and defenseless.

The drug companies pride themselves in the fact that each batch of the drug is a specific chemical makeup and the same in each batch manufactured. These drugs do the exact thing year after year and because of this the bacteria learn how to recognize it and adapt in ways that protect them and make them resistant to it over time.

This is what makes all antibacterial useless over time. The intelligence of the bacteria win eventually over the drug.

The endless variation of a specific oil is considered a liability to the druggists, but it is the most advantageous quality of an essential oil. A resistance to an essential oil has never been known to happen because oils that were effective thousands of years ago in Egypt are just as effective today as they were then.

When bacteria become resistant to the most potent and powerful antibiotic then the use of antibiotics will be over. We need to look for alternatives and the best alternatives are essential oils.

Many essential oils fight bacteria and will never develop resistance. They also have another advantage. They can fight viruses as well as bacteria.

Many people now know that essential oils fight viral infections that we are more prone to during the cold and flu season.

These people need no studies to tell them they work.

Their experience is enough proof for them.

CHAPTER NINE

INTELLIGENT OILS VS. NON-INTELLIGENT DRUGS

Our bodies function the best with the help of millions of friendly bacteria that live in our intestines. When antibiotics are used they kill everything – the good and the bad bacteria.

The fragrant essential oils know the difference between bacteria we need and invaders to our bodies. They kill the invaders and leave the friendly bacteria alone. They are made by our magnificent God and embedded with His gracious intelligence. When using antibiotics, we are left in a very weakened condition. Our whole system is compromised and susceptible to the next germ that comes along.

When using essential oils our system becomes stronger and able to deal with the next round of disease-causing germs.

Antibiotics can seem to work faster than the oils but in the long run they also do you harm. Usually it is not long before you get the same illness.

When using the medicine created by God, the oils and herbs, there are usually no negative side effects. Many times when using the oils to correct one problem, another problem disappears as well.

CHAPTER TEN

QUICKNESS VS. SAFETY

I am not saying that antibiotics have no place. In a real emergency, a shot of antibiotics may save your life and give your body a short term advantage

 When using essential oils, it might act too slowly.

Please consult a licensed health care provider when a decision like that is needed. There are times when antibiotics are needed.

True healing comes from another source.

CHAPTER ELEVEN

QUICK REFERENCE GUIDE FOR SOME COMMON ESSENTIAL OILS

ESSENTIAL OIL	USES
Cinnamon aches	Toothaches, body
Clove fungus	memory support,
Lavender relaxation	Swelling, sleep,
Lemon swelling	stomach aches, joint
Peppermint health	dizziness, digestive

Rosemary	memory support, joint aches
Spearmint	nerves, blemishes, cramps
Tangerine	age spots, water retention
Tea Tree	cold sores, swollen glands
Ylang Ylang	fear, healthy skin, nerves

CHAPTER TWELVE

THE TRUE CERTIFIED ORGANIC ESSENTIAL OILS

Many companies say that their oils are natural, pure, clean or therapeutic yet not tested for quality outside of their own company. If it is not 100% Organic and tested for purity by independent inspectors not the companies themselves and certified to be organic it isn't.

If you want the 100% Organic Essential Oils, contact me at: cynthia.forck279@gmail.com or on Facebook on my page:

https://www.facebook.com/cynthia.forck

or feel free to private message me. I am here for you!

The FDA has not evaluated these statements. Products are not intended to diagnose, treat, cure or prevent disease.